Book 1
Thyroid Diet

BY LINDSEY P

&

Book 2
The Beginners Guide to Medicinal Plants

BY LINDSEY P

Book 1
Thyroid Diet
BY LINDSEY P

Easy Guide to Managing Thyroid Symptoms, Losing Weight, Increasing Your Metabolism

Essential Oils Box Set #40: Thyroid Diet & The Beginners Guide to Medicinal Plants

Table Of Contents

Introduction

I want to thank you and congratulate you for purchasing the book, *"Thyroid Diet: Easy Guide To Managing Thyroid Symptoms, Losing Weight, Increasing Your Metabolism"*

This book contains proven steps and strategies on how to take care of your thyroid gland. This small gland located in the neck drives the body's metabolism. Imbalance of the hormonal functions would mean disturbances in different aspects of the body, like digestion, weight control and energy. Even sleep can get affected, too.

In this book, learn all about the thyroid gland, its hormones, its functions and how you can keep it healthy. A healthy organ is a healthy body. Learn about how the thyroid function can go off balance. Know about the different disorders related to it, the causes and how these can be managed.

Also, learn about the thyroid diet- what is it, what can it do and how you can use it for yourself. There are a lot of things you need to learn about your body. Start with your thyroid.

Thanks again for purchasing this book, I hope you enjoy it!

Chapter 1 Your Thyroid

Each and every organ in the body, big or small, plays an important role in the body. Each function is an integral part of a whole complex of chemical and metabolic processes that keep the body in homeostasis. One of the small organs with huge important function is the thyroid gland.

Located in front of the neck, the thyroid gland sits just below the Adam's apple and in front of the windpipe. It has a butterfly shape, each "wing" is a lobe connected to each other via an isthmus located between them. This gland is normally brownish red from the rich blood supply from its abundant blood vessels.

The thyroid gland is about 2 inches big. It is composed of 2 cell types, namely, the follicular and the parafollicular cells. The follicular cells make up most of the thyroid tissues. These cells are responsible in secreting the hormones thyroxine (T4) and triiodothyronine (T3). On the other hand, parafollicular cells are responsible for the secretion of another thyroid hormone called calcitonin.

Thyroid Gland Function

The main function of the thyroid gland is to regulate the metabolism and calcium balance in the body. This function is carried out by the various thyroid hormones. The T3 and T4 hormones regulate metabolism. Calcitonin helps in maintaining calcium balance.

The signal to start and stop thyroid hormone synthesis and secretion comes from the thyroid-stimulating hormone secreted by the pituitary gland. The hypothalamus, in turn, sends a signal to the pituitary gland to regulate the signaling mechanism.

Thyroid Hormones

Three basic thyroid hormones work with the rest of the body in order to maintain homeostasis. These hormones are T3, T4 and calcitonin. T4 and T3 are considered as the main thyroid hormones, as they carry out the

T4 and T3 hormones are produced by the follicular cells of the thyroid gland. Iodine plays an important role in the production of these 2 hormones.

T3 and T4 stimulate the various cells in the body. They promote protein synthesis and increase the rate of cellular oxygen consumption. In absence of these hormones, the body cannot breakdown and metabolizes proteins, vitamins and carbohydrates.

T3 and T4 work together to influence other endocrine glands, as well. They influence the production and release of adrenaline and epinephrine. T3 and T4 also play a role in dopamine production and secretion in the brain.

Essential Oils Box Set #40: Thyroid Diet & The Beginners Guide to Medicinal Plants

The thyroid makes sure that there is adequate, steady and ready supply of T3 and T4 in the body. A few "droplets" of these hormones are stored within the thyroid gland, ready for release once TSH (thyroid stimulating hormone) sends a signal for their release and activation. Some of T3 and T4 are bound to carrier proteins and circulate in the blood. This is why blood tests can reveal if there are sufficient thyroid hormones in the body.

If the body needs thyroid hormones at any given time, the carrier proteins free the bound T3 and T4 hormones. These hormones would then travel to the cells that need them and work their effect.

Together, T3 and T4 increase the body's basal metabolic rate. That would mean the following bodily responses:

- Rise in body temperature

- Stronger _heartbeat_

- increased pulse

- Faster digestion and use of ingested food

- Faster utilization of energy resources stored in the muscles and liver

- Promotes brain maturation in children

- Growth promotion in children

- Activation of the nervous system, causing better levels of attention and Better reflex action

Calcitonin hormone plays a role in maintaining calcium balance in the body. It works together with hormones produced by another gland called the parathyroid glands. The C-cells within the thyroid gland synthesize this hormone. It plays vital roles in calcium regulation and bone metabolism.

Chapter 2 Thyroid Imbalance

Thyroid gland function can become compromised, leading to inadequate circulating and stored hormones. Imbalances in thyroid hormone production can affect all aspects of body function, which includes weight regulation, control and regulation of other hormones, digestion process, live function, and a whole lot more.

Causes of Thyroid Problems

There are basically two types of thyroid imbalance- hyper and hypo. Hyperthyroidism means the thyroid gland is producing more hormones than necessary. Hypothyroidism means the thyroid gland is not producing adequate amounts of hormones.

Hyperthyroidism is caused by the following:

- Graves' disease

  This is a result of overproduction of thyroid hormones.

- Toxic adenomas

  Sometimes, nodules grow in the thyroid. These nodules can secrete thyroid hormones that can upset the hormonal balance. Some goiters have nodules that have hormone-secreting capacity.

- Subacute thyroiditis

  This is an inflammatory condition of the thyroid gland. The inflammation causes the stored thyroid hormones to leak out of the gland and into the blood. This will cause an increase in the amounts of circulating thyroid hormones, leading to hyperthyroidism. In this case, hyperthyroidism may be temporary, lasting for a few weeks to a few months. Generally, the hormonal imbalance will resolve on its own after the thyroid gland inflammation subsides.

- Malfunctioning pituitary gland

  The pituitary gland sends the signal for thyroid hormone production. More pituitary gland signaling means more thyroid hormone production. Sometimes, tumors and other pituitary problems can cause more signals sent for thyroid hormone synthesis leading to hyperthyroidism.

Hypothyroidism is too little production of thyroid hormones. This would cause too little energy for metabolic processes. Common causes of hypothyroidism include:

- Hashimoto's thyroiditis

This is an autoimmune disease attacks and destroys the cells in the thyroid glands. The thyroid cells eventually die, causing the gland to produce less hormones.

- Thyroid gland removal

  Destruction and removal of the thyroid gland may cause inadequate hormone production. This may be due to surgical removal or chemical destruction.

- Excessive exposure to iodide

  Hypothyroidism may also be caused by too much exposure to iodine. This may come from use of contrast dyes, sinus and cold medicines, and cardiac medicines such as amiodarone.

- Lithium

  In some individuals, taking lithium has been found to cause a decrease in the circulating thyroid hormones.

Signs and Symptoms of Thyroid Problems

Thyroid problems may manifest in a wide range of symptoms. The most common ones are the following:

- Fatigue

  This is the most common symptom of thyroid problems. It may be vague but it is the most commonly experienced symptom. A person wakes up feeling tired despite getting adequate amounts if sleep. All throughout the day, the need to nap is very common. Also, people with hyperthyroidism have difficulty falling asleep or maintaining a restful sleep.

- Weight changes

  Weight is heavily influenced by thyroid hormones. Often, difficulty losing weight despite low-fat and calorie diets coupled with rigorous exercise is a sign of hypothyroidism. Unintentional weight loss despite no changes in the amount of consumed food is a sign of hyperthyroidism.

- Heat intolerance

  People with hyperthyroidism would often feel warmer than usual.

- Feels cold easily

  Hypothyroidism causes a person to feel cold all the time, with no relation at all to weather or room temperature.

- Pain in the muscles and joints

9

Thyroid hormones influence calcium and energy consumption by the bones and muscles. Often, thyroid problems can cause muscle and joint aches and pains. It may also cause weakness in the muscles and joints that can further develop into carpal tunnel syndrome (in the hands or arms), tarsal tunnel syndrome (in the legs) and plantar fasciitis in the feet.

- Discomfort or enlargement of the neck

Thyroid enlargement may cause outward signs such as swelling or enlargement in the neck area. It may also be manifested as discomfort when wearing something over the neck such as scarves and neckties.

- Changes in the hair and/or skin

The hair and the skin are sensitive to changes in the thyroid function. Hypothyroidism would often cause the hair to become dry, coarse, and brittle breaks off and falls easily. It can also cause the outer edge of the eyebrows to fall off. The skin becomes dry, thick, scaly and coarse.

Hyperthyroidism can cause severe hair loss. The skin becomes thin and fragile, causing it to become injured easily.

- Changes in the bowel function

Thyroid hormones influence other systems as well. Problems in the thyroid function can also cause changes in the functioning of other systems. In the digestive system, hypothyroidism can cause severe or chronic constipation. Hyperthyroidism can cause IBS (irritable bowel syndrome) or frequent diarrhea.

- Reproductive changes

Women who have thyroid problems often experience irregularities in their menstrual periods. Hyperthyroidism is often associated with infrequent periods. Menstruation is often of short duration with lighter flow. Hypothyroidism causes menstrual periods to occur more often. Flow is often heavier and more painful.

Fertility is also affected by thyroid imbalance. There may be infertility concerns in both men and women.

- Cholesterol problems

High cholesterol levels unresponsive to diet, medication and exercise are often associated with hypothyroidism. Very low cholesterol that is unusual may be signifying hyperthyroidism.

- Mental changes

Essential Oils Box Set #40: Thyroid Diet & The Beginners Guide to Medicinal Plants

Hypothyroidism is often associated with depression. Hyperthyroidism is associated with panic or anxiety attacks.

- Tremors and nervousness

  Hyperthyroidism causes muscle tremors, agitation and nervousness.

- Bloated

  From fluid retention due to hypothyroidism

- Tachycardia and palpitations

Chapter 3 Restoring Balance through Diet

Nutrition plays an important role in regulating thyroid function. A lot of nutrients can increase or decrease this gland's function. Some improve the cell susceptibility to thyroid hormones. Some are used as part of the hormone synthesis process.

Iodine

This is the single most important nutrient for thyroid health. The hormones T3 and T4 rely on the presence of iodine for production. One of the main causes of thyroid dysfunction is due to iodine deficiency.

The body has no capacity to manufacture this trace element. It needs to be obtained from dietary sources. Iodine from food is released through the digestive process. It is then absorbed by the intestines and brought to the blood stream. The blood then brings iodine to the thyroid glands, where it becomes part of thyroid hormone production.

Major source of iodine is iodized salt. This fortified salt ensures that people will be getting the recommended daily amounts of this very important trace mineral. Other sources include grains, fish and dairy.

Iodine supplements are one of the options for treating deficiencies and improving thyroid function. However, excess iodine can cause thyroid imbalance and other problems, too. People with Hashimoto's disease may experience flare-ups with iodine supplements.

Vitamin D

A study showed that Hashimoto's disease and vitamin D deficiency are linked. About 90% of patients with this form of thyroid disorder have been found to be deficient in vitamin D.

Patients with Grave's disease also suffer from bone loss. Vitamin D worsens bone loss in this disorder. The loss of bone mass often resolves as thyroid condition improves. Experts agree that it can also be treated by giving vitamin D supplements, especially before and after thyroid treatments.

Food sources rich in vitamin D include milk, dairy, eggs, mushrooms and fatty fish. Supplemental vitamin D3 is also given to some patients. While on supplemental D3, the patient needs to be constantly monitored to ensure that the vitamin D levels should be within the desired therapeutic range.

Selenium

Selenium in the body is concentrated in the thyroid gland. This mineral is a component of important enzymes that influence thyroid function. Also, it has been found that selenium can affect cognitive function, immune system, mortality and fertility in both men and women.

Studies have found that selenium boosts the levels of circulating thyroid hormones. It also improves the mood of people suffering from Hashimoto's disease.

On the other hand, excessive selenium intake can cause health problems such as gastrointestinal upset. Too much selenium can also increase the risk for type 2 diabetes and some cancers.

Selenium levels should be constantly monitored while on supplements and treatment. Selenium-rich foods are less likely to cause serious side effects. Good food sources include tuna, Brazil nuts, lobster and crabs.

Vitamin B12

Studies made among people with thyroid disorders have found that about 30% also suffer from vitamin B12 deficiency. Severe deficiency with this vitamin is irreversible and having a thyroid disorder can worsen the problem. Supplement with food sources like seafood such as salmon, sardines and mollusks. Other great sources of vitamin B12 include dairy, lean meats and organ meats such as the liver. Plant sources of vitamin B12 include nutritional yeast and fortified cereals.

Goitrogens

Goitrogens are foods that have been found to interfere with thyroid hormone synthesis. The active compound in these foods is called goitrin. This compound is released when the food is hydrolyzed. However, goitrin only becomes a concern if there is an existing iodine deficiency state in the body. Also, goitrin is easily denatured (destroyed or inactivated) and the goitrogenic effects rendered ineffective when is heated. Well-known goitrogenic foods are the cruciferous vegetables like cauliflower, cabbage and broccoli.

Aside from cruciferous vegetables, soy is also a potential goitrogen. Soy contains the compounds isoflavones, which can slow down the rate of thyroid hormone synthesis. However, soy does not directly cause hypothyroidism. The isoflavones do not cause profound thyroid imbalance if there are good iodine stores in the body.

Millet is another potential goitrogen. This gluten-free, nutritious grain has been found to affect thyroid function. People with adequate iodine stores experience suppression of their thyroid function when consuming millet. People suffering from hypothyroidism are especially advised to avoid taking millet.

Medications and Supplements

Some medications and supplements have been found to affect thyroid function. Calcium supplements may help with reducing bone loss, but can interfere with the absorption of thyroid medications. In order to harness the benefits of calcium supplements and reduce the interference with thyroid medications, patients are advised to take these separately. Experts advise waiting at least 4 hours in between taking calcium supplements and thyroid medications.

Fiber supplements and coffee have also been found to lower the rate of absorption of thyroid medication. In order to decrease the interference from these foods, take them at least 1 hour apart.

Another compound that interferes with thyroid function and thyroid medication is chromium picolinate. This compound is marketed for weight loss and blood sugar control. Taking chromium picolinate lowers thyroid hormone function and interferes with thyroid medication action. Take them at least 3 to 4 hours apart.

Fruits, green tea and vegetables contain beneficial flavonoids that have great health benefits. They improve cardiovascular health and helps in preventing several serious illnesses like stroke and cancers. However, studies have shown that taking large amounts of flavonoids, especially in supplemental forms, suppress the action of thyroid hormones. Experts recommend consulting a dietician and physician in order to get a balance of flavonoid benefits and thyroid function.

Chapter 4 Thyroid Diet

In order to help return the balance and normal function of the thyroid gland, experts have formulated the thyroid diet. The aim of this diet is to

Thyroid diet is an individualized diet that aims to provide the necessary nutrients the body needs while improving thyroid function. To start, calculate the calories needed by the body on a daily basis. Then make adjustments depending on the desired outcome of the thyroid diet.

Calories

To get the daily caloric needs:

1. Get the current body weight in kilograms. If using pounds, convert the weight to kilograms by dividing the value by 2.2.

   Thus, for a person weighing 165 pounds, convert it to kilograms by dividing it by 2.2, which will yield 75 kilograms.

2. Multiply the weight (in kilograms) by 30. The number 30 refers to the number of calories the body needs for each pound of body weight.

   For the same person above, multiply the weight of 75 kilograms by 30, which is 2250. So, theoretically, a person weighing 75 kilograms needs 2250 calories in a day.

3. From the computed daily calorie needs, subtract 200. This is an estimation that reflects the need to reduce the calorie intake in relation to the thyroid condition.

   Therefore, a person who weighs 75 kilograms needs 2250 calories in a day. Because of a thyroid condition, less calories is needed in order to maintain the same 75-kilogram weight. Hence, in order to maintain the current weight, the person with a thyroid condition needs 2050 calories in a day.

4. If the goal of going on a thyroid diet is to lose weight, the daily calorie requirements should be reduced by 5 calories for each kilogram of body weight. That would be multiplying the weight in kilograms by 25 instead of 30.

   So, a person who weighs 75 kilograms and wants to lose weight using the thyroid diet would multiply the weight by 25 instead of 30. That will be 1875 calories per day. This, in theory, is the daily calorie need in order to lose 1 pound of body weight every 10 days.

Then subtract the 200 calories to account for the thyroid condition. Thus, a person weighing 75 kilograms who has a thyroid condition and wants to use the thyroid diet for weight loss would need to take 1675 calories per day in order to lose weight safely.

Pillars of the Thyroid Diet

The thyroid diet is formulated based on the following basic concepts:

I. Protecting the thyroid from harmful substances

Most thyroid imbalances are caused by the destruction or damage to the thyroid gland. Inflammation causes hormones to leak out into the blood, cellular destruction can cause low hormone production. Remove substances that are detrimental to thyroid health.

a. Sugar

Fluctuations in the sugar levels can cause hormones to go off balance, including the thyroid hormones. If there is sugar imbalance in the body, thyroid function will a take a long time to improve. This is because the pancreas that regulates sugar metabolism also affects thyroid function.

Limit daily sugar intake to no more than 5 spoons. In 1 teaspoon of sugar, there are 4 grams of sugar. In a tablespoon, 12 grams of sugar is present.

Combat sugar cravings by eating a high protein, high fat breakfast. Energy from these foods will help tide the body over until lunch, which completely avoids the mid-morning energy and sugar crash that leads to cravings.

b. Food Intolerances

Most people experience thyroid disturbances when eating gluten-containing foods. Eliminating it from the diet has shown improvement in their thyroid conditions. Also, it may be necessary to eliminate more than gluten it usually needs to eliminate the big 5- foods that are common causes of food intolerances. The big 5 are gluten, soy, dairy, eggs and corn.

c. Improve gut health

The gut or the digestive system plays an important role in managing thyroid disorders. A huge concentration of immune cells such as lymphocytes is present in the gut. Imbalance in this part would often cause autoimmune disorders, one of the leading causes of thyroid dysfunction.

d. Avoid toxic substances

Avoid foods that contain toxic ingredients such as preservatives, additives, excessive sodium, artificial sweeteners and trans fats. Also, avoid exposure to environmental toxins from house cleaners and other substances.

Water toxicity has been found to be an increasing contributing factor to thyroid problems. Fluoride in water has been linked to hypothyroidism. This element has been found to enter the thyroid gland and reduce iodine uptake. Decreased uptake of iodine means slowed production of T4 thyroid hormone.

e. Detoxify

T4 hormone is inactive and needs to be converted into active T3 in order to work its effects on the body. Conversion happens in the liver and the digestive tract. Sluggish liver and gut means slow conversion of thyroid hormones. Detoxify to keep these organs in top shape.

f. Manage stress and adrenal fatigue

Thyroid and adrenal function are closely linked. Managing thyroid means managing adrenals. Stress fires up the adrenals and cause adrenal fatigue. This will cause thyroid function to slow down. De-stress to reduce strain on the adrenals and also ease up on the thyroid.

g. Goitrous foods

Goiter slows down the function of the thyroid gland. Goitrogenic food can worsen goiter, which can cause hypothyroidism. Avoid goitrous foods like Brussels, sprouts, bok choy, cauliflower, mustard greens, broccoli, and other cruciferous vegetables. Also, avoid soy, tofu and lecithin.

II. Consume more foods that promote healing thyroid

a. Foods that are paced with macro- and micro-nutrients

Choose organic, hormone-free foods. The growth hormones fed to meats and poultry can interrupt the normal function of the endocrine system.

b. Protein and fat

Proteins and fats are the backbones of the body's hormones. Eat them in the right proportions and from the right sources. Choose healthy fat sources such as fish and seafood oil, olive oil and coconut oil. Also, eat foods that are naturally rich in healthy fats such as avocados and coconuts. Good protein sources are from lean cuts of meats, poultry without the skin on and from beans.

c. Probiotics

Probiotics help restore the balance of good bacteria in the gut. Good bacteria help in preventing the absorption of bad compounds and toxins from the gut and into the blood. Add probiotics to the diet by eating foods that have naturally fermented. Examples are:

- Kim chee (Korean fermented veggies)

- Sauerkraut (not fermented in vinegar)

- Yoghurt

- Kombucha tea

- Kefir

- Coconut water

- Vegetable medley (fermented)

d. Herbs and supplements

Get the recommended daily dose of vitamins and minerals such as vitamin D, calcium and selenium.

e. Meditation

f. Exercise

Exercise helps to restart the hormone balance. It also helps in better circulation of hormones and better cellular response.

III. Balance according to the body's needs

Everyone has unique health needs. Cater to the individual needs by taking into consideration all the individual's needs according to age, height, weight, activity and overall health condition.

Chapter 5 Thyroid Diet Food Guide

Certain foods contain compounds that can influence thyroid function. There are foods that can improve thyroid levels. Some foods interfere with thyroid function. People should learn what foods help thyroid in functioning normally and which foods to avoid that can interfere with the thyroid glands.

Foods to eat

Avocado and potato

These foods are rich in amino acid tyrosine. Studies have found that low tyrosine level is linked to hypothyroidism.

Artichokes

Artichokes have powerful detoxifying effect on the liver. Clear liver means better at producing proteins that can bind and carry thyroid hormones for circulation in the blood.

Sea vegetables

These are notoriously rich in iodine, which a main component of thyroid hormone synthesis. Good ones include arame, kombu, kelp, dulse and wakame.

Beans

Beans contain an abundance of iodine. Aside from this trace mineral, beans are also good sources of fiber. The fiber helps to relieve constipation that most people with hypothyroidism suffer from.

Foods rich in Iodine (good for hypothyroidism)

- Iodized Salt
- Seaweeds and Seafoods
- Celtic Sea Salt
- Salt Water Fish
- Nori Rolls
- Sushi

Foods rich in Selenium (good for hypothyroidism)

- Meat
- Salmon

- Chicken

- Tuna

- Brazil Nuts

- Whole Unrefined Grains

- Dairy Products

- Onions

- Garlic

Herbs

Herbs help to boost the metabolism. Some help in detoxifying the body, such as cilantro, which removes mercury that is toxic to the thyroid gland.

- Black Pepper

- Tumeric

- Chilies

- Ginger

- Garlic

- Cinnamon

- Peppermint

- Parsley

- Cilantro

- Rosemary

Fruits

Fruits contain trace minerals such as iodine and selenium. They also contain antioxidants that detoxify the body and boost overall bodily function.

Cranberries, in particular, are rich in iodine. About 400 mcg (micrograms) of iodine is contained in ½ cup of this fruit.

Other thyroid-friendly fruits are:

- Apples

- Apricots

- Bananas

- Blueberries

- Blackberries

- Cherries

- Cranberries

- Dates

- Grapefruit

- Kiwi

- Papaya

- Pineapple

- Prunes

- Raspberries

Grains

Grains help to regulate sugar levels that can otherwise put off sugar balance. Good grains include:

- Amaranth

- Quinoa

- Buckwheat

- Brown Rice

- Wild Rice

Oils

Good oils are great fat sources, which the thyroid can use to synthesize thyroid hormones. Coconut oil, in particular, stimulates the thyroid gland to increase hormone production. Olive oil and raw butter also have good effects on thyroid function.

Foods to avoid (which can worsen hypothyroidism)

While foods can help stimulate better thyroid function, some foods have known negative effects on this gland. Avoid the following, which are detrimental to thyroid health:

- Cassava
- Kohlrabi
- Linseed
- Turnips
- Kale
- Peanuts
- Mustard
- Mustard Greens
- Cauliflower
- Millet
- Rutabagas
- Spinach
- Peaches
- Coffee

Goitrogenic foods

- Soybeans and related products
- Bamboo shoots
- Canola Oil
- Bok Choy
- Horseradish
- Sweet Potato
- Foods with Gluten
- Tempeh
- Garden Kres
- Babassu

Goitrogenic Chemicals

Essential Oils Box Set #40: Thyroid Diet & The Beginners Guide to Medicinal Plants

- Lithium
- Amiodarone
- Carbamazepine
- Oxazolidines
- Minocycline (MN)
- Iopanoic acid
- Thioureylene
- Propylthiouracil
- Sulfadimethoxine
- Phenobarbitone

Chapter 6 Thyroid Diet for Weight Loss

As has been previously mentioned, people can use the thyroid diet for weight loss. People suffering from hypothyroidism are the main reasons for this weight loss diet. Hypothyroidism can cause weight gain. In order to lose weight or at least maintain it at a normal level, experts advise using the specially formulated thyroid diet.

The most effective weight loss program designed for thyroid patients focuses not only on calorie counts but also on spacing caloric intake throughout the day. That is, the calculated calorie intake is taken in several mini-meals.

Also, experts believe that people who suffer from hypothyroidism need to adjust the proportions and distribution of macronutrient intake. That is, a meal should comprise of 40% proteins, 35% carbohydrates (from low glycemic index foods), and 25% fats, with 250 to 300 calories at each meal.

Let's take a closer look into the previous example:

A person who weighs 75 kilograms (165 pounds) with a thyroid condition (e.g., hypothyroidism) wants to lose weight safely.

Get the daily calorie needs: 75 kilograms X 25 = 1875 calories per day

Subtract 200 calories (thyroid factor, to account for thyroid condition):

> 1875-200= 1675 calories per day for safe weight loss

Divide a day's worth of meals into mini-meals, with 300 calories each meal. To get the number of 300-calorie meals per day, divide the calorie for weight loss by 300:

> 1675 calories / 300 = 5.58 or 6 mini-meals a day

This means that a person who weighs 75 kilograms would need to eat 6 mini meals each day, at 300 calories per meal in order to lose weight safely. The mini-meals should be evenly spaced out throughout the day.

The recommended rate of weight loss is at 1 kilogram or 2.2 pounds a week only. Going more than that can trigger starvation mode in the body. While the body still has adequate fat and energy stores, abruptly and severely reducing food intake will cause the body to recognize it as going into starvation. Instead of losing weight and burning fats, the body tries really hard to retain all the fats and to keep eating. Cravings will o over the top in this case, which can lead to serious overeating and gaining back more weight than what was initially lost.

So, in order to lose weight effectively and sustainably, lose weight gradually and safely.

Conclusion

Thank you again for purchasing this book!

I hope this book was able to help you to learn more about the thyroid gland, the disorders, and how these can be managed. The thyroid diet is an affective diet both for restoring thyroid health and in losing weight.

The next step is to start making that healthier choice. Start making the changes today and live a healthier life. The changes may be difficult at first but with solid determination to become a healthier person, it will all be worth it. Also, share with family and friends about this wonderful book and the knowledge it imparts. Get them to accompany you in this health journey and experience the health benefits of the thyroid diet.

Finally, if you enjoyed this book, please take the time to share your thoughts and post a review on Amazon. We do our best to reach out to readers and provide the best value we can. Your positive review will help us achieve that. It'd be greatly appreciated!

Thank you and good luck!

Book 2
The Beginners Guide to Medicinal Plants

BY LINDSEY P

Everything You Need to Know About the Healing Properties of Plants & Herbs, How to Grow and Harvest Them

Essential Oils Box Set #40: Thyroid Diet & The Beginners Guide to Medicinal Plants

Table Of Contents

Introduction

I want to thank you and congratulate you for purchasing the book, *"The Beginners Guide to Medicinal Plants"*.

This book contains proven steps and strategies on how to successfully grow medicinal plants and herbs right at the very comfort of your own home.

Featured in this book are some of the most common mistakes when putting up a medicinal garden at home and how to avoid committing such mistakes. Also featured in this book are some of the best types of medicinal plants to grow at home.

Thanks again for purchasing this book, I hope you enjoy it!

Chapter 1: Guide to Growing a Medicinal Herb Garden

Growing medicinal plants and herbs indoor is a popular hobby for a lot of gardeners. One of the greatest reasons to plant medicinal plants indoor is to have a ready supply of these beneficial herbs. These herbs are those that you commonly snip into your sauces and soups. They can also be used to soothe an itchy rash or cough. Growing medicinal herbs may not sound to be very appealing, however you can benefit from growing these plants that can provide instant relief for many illnesses that can happen anytime of the day.

It would also be wonderful to be able to cut a sprig of thyme while boiling water and prepare a fresh cup of thyme tea that is fragrant and vibrant. Since it is fresh, you'll sure it is effective since it's fresh.

So what kind of medicinal plants should you grow? The next chapter of this book features a list of different herbs and medicinal plants that you can grow at home. The list is just a good starting point for easy to find and easy to grow herbs. The same plants that you can use in cooking daily may also be used as teas, salves, washes and tinctures. You can also make cough syrup and cough drops with the very same herbal plants that you grow in the comforts of your own home.

No matter how you thoroughly care for your medicinal plants, in the long run, they will have to be replaced. If this should happen during the colder days, you will have to take into account the growing time, before they will be big enough for harvest. Commonly, this will take about 4 to 6 weeks. You can make use of these herbs not only for cooking but for medicinal purposes as well.

What problems can you possibly encounter while growing medicinal plants and herbs in your home garden? While herbs typically suffer from much less issues that flowers and vegetables do, there are a few things that should be looked out for. Plants grown in your home garden may also encounter some basic problems such as molds or mildew problems, insect damage and most of all, fertilizer issues. To remedy these problems, you must know the following guidelines:

1. Home Garden Temperature

    While most of us think our homes as a temperate area would be ideal for growing plants, this is not always the case.

    A plant requires light in order to make food, a process which we know as photosynthesis. While plants are very adaptable, they grow best within a 70 to 75 degree range. A plant utilizes more energy when the temperature is warm than when it is cold. Plants can adapt to a cooler room, for instance, with an air conditioner. The plants will begin the process of photosynthesis with the increase in temperature and there will be no sunlight to produce food. When this happens, the plants will not most likely to thrive and will probably die.

So what is the best temperature for growing medicinal herbs?

Plants grow best when there is at least a 10 degree fall in temperature during the night. During the summer, the temperature tends to get high and stay high. Plants get stressed and become highly susceptible to diseases. They grow less and can drop leaves, weaken and die, despite sufficient watering. If you are growing herbs indoors, it would be a good idea to grow them around a room based on available temperature zones. Save a lot of money and be stress-free by working on with what you already have instead of trying to make big modifications that work against the natural rhythm of your home environment.

2. Home Garden Fertilizer

Once you have already decided on which type of herbs that you will grow in your home garden, you will now have to choose the most suitable fertilizer for them. Not all fertilizers are created the same. While most have advertising claims, these fertilizers may be overused enough to damage your medicinal herbs grown at home.

What kinds of fertilizers can be used at home? There are a lot of fertilizer types that will work for your medicinal herb garden at home. For indoor plants, you can try using a variety that can be dissolved in water (water-soluble). This particular type of fertilizer may come in packaged granular form that you measure and dissolve in water prior to application. It may also come in the form of a fish emulsion, which is a concentrated variety and is combined with water before application.

Regardless on the type of fertilizer that you choose to use, you must apply it at one quarter of the packaging's recommended amount. Apply this light mixture once every week. For a more effective application, make sure to water your plants thoroughly and then apply the prepared fertilizer solution. This technique will allow for better absorption by the plant.

More importantly, make sure that you do a monthly flushing of your medicinal plants. This can be done by placing the plant in a sink and water entirely, allowing the excess water to draw off. Once the dripping stops, water completely once again. This technique will get rid of any salts that may have accumulated in the plant's soil.

31

Chapter 2: Easy Guide to Successfully Grow Herbs and Medicinal Plants at Home

Follow this easy step-by-step guide to start with your medicinal herb garden at home:

1. Choose your herbs. When growing medicinal herbs at home, it is important to have a good variety of herbs as well as companion plants. Some of the good choice include the following:

   - Hot pepper
   - Strawberries
   - Oregano
   - Thyme
   - Lime basil
   - Mint
   - Common basil
   - Sage
   - Lemon balm
   - Sweet marjoram

2. Prepare your pot. Be sure that the pots that you will be using for your medicinal plants have holes at the bottom to provide good drainage. With a grit or gravel, pour to about a quarter of the pot's depth. This will allow the water to steep out from the soil's bottom.

3. Fill. When the gravel is already in place, begin to fill the pot with soil-based or multi-purpose compost. Fill t about three (3) quarters of the pot's remaining space.

4. Begin planting – put the medicinal plants into the pot, with around 15 centimeters between each stem. Squeeze every plant lightly from its temporary pot. To encourage the plants to spread out, tease the roots from the root ball.

5. Put the trailing plants near the edge and the taller ones in the center of the display. This technique will endure the best growth for your plants. DO not worry if the display may seem to appear messy at first. This will begin to fill out and look lush in just a few weeks.

6. Fill in the spaces around the plants. When you are already satisfied with the positions, begin filling in the gaps in between the plants with compost. Tightly push the compost into the spaces by pushing your fingers deep into the soil. Be careful not to injure the roots. Add more if needed. To avoid overflowing when being waters, leave a few centimeters between the rim of the pot and the soil.

7. Top the plants. Cut the taller plants' top. This will encourage them to bush out and give more fresh leaves to pick during harvest time.

8. Fertilize regularly. Purchase a controlled release fertilizer which should last a whole season. This will mean that you won't have to feed the pot again.

9. Water. Water your plants thoroughly or until the water begins to drain out of the pot's bottom. Medicinal plants usually like to dry out between watering and some types of medicinal plants such as Rosemary can easily be over-watered.

Growing herbs and medicinal plants at home is an easy yet a very rewarding hobby. Below are seven (7) key steps that will surely help you to successfully grow a healthy medicinal herb at home:

1. Keep an eye on Pests

   Medicinal herbs are generally not bothered so much about pests as much as flowers and vegetables can be. In an indoor garden however, the non-natural conditions may increase the possibility of a pest problem. To keep pests from damaging your medicinal plants in your indoor garden, make sure to keep a close eye. At the very first sight of infestation, make use of a soapy spray. You may also handpick any pests that you may have come to notices and put sticky traps to get rid of the rest.

2. Water your plants regularly

   Medicinal herbs require thorough attention when it comes to watering. Whether your medicinal plants likes drier conditions or extra moisture, it is never a good idea to have plants to be sitting in water.

3. Apply fertilizer

   Always keep in mind that medicinal plants grown indoors require a special fertilization schedule than those which are planted in an outdoor environment.

4. Be mindful of the soil

Indoor gardening soil needs to have effective exceptional drainage. It also needs to be light. Whether your medicinal plants like drier conditions or with extra moisture, having your plants to sit in water is never a good idea. Specifically buy potting soil. You may also prepare your own by using a part of peat moss, a part of sand and a part of bagged potting soil.

5. Ensure proper circulation

Medicinal plants require sufficient airflow to keep pests and bacterial organisms at bay. Just make sure to keep the air moving in the area where you will grow your medicinal plants.

6. Check your temperature

Keep your planting area at constant temperature. The ideal temperature for a home garden is about 60 to 70 degrees.

7. Provide enough light

Provide about 14 to 16 hours of artificial light to keep your medicinal plants healthy. You can also alternatively expose them to natural light for about 6 hours a day.

Chapter 3: The Best Medicinal Plants to Grow at Home

Do you have a small space at home to grow some plants? Why not grow some medicinal plants? Growing your own medicinal plants will not only get a lot of enjoyment but this will also provide medicinal relief at the comforts of your own home. While herbal remedies must never take the place of professional health care, it would be nice to have a sense of self-help should you ever end up having to need instant relief. Below is a list of the best plants to start your own personal medicinal plants garden:

1. Echinacea – this herb is also popularly known as the purple coneflower. Echinacea is an American perennial wildflower which is popularly known for its stimulating effects in the immune system. Preparations made with this wonder herb are used for the treatment of flu, colds, minor infections and a wide range of various illnesses.

2. Lavender – is medicinal plant which is commonly used as a fragrance these days. Lavender has been widely used since ancient times to reduce swelling, provide relief for rashes and itching and to treat burns, bug bites and other skin orders.

3. Lemon Balm – Prepare potent lemonade by adding bruised lemon balm leaves into your drink. This herb is commonly used as a calming "night tea" to combat insomnia. It can also make an effective topical relief for cold sores.

4. Comfrey – The roots of this wonder herb are cooked and mashed to make a potent topical relief for sprains, burns, bruises and arthritis. Just do not eat it. There is a study which reported that this herb can potentially damage the liver in eaten in significant amounts.

5. St. John's Wort – this wonder herb can lift the mood very well that you must keep from using this when you are already taking other forms of anti-depressants. The flowers and leaves of this herb may be used to prepare a tea. They can also be soaked in liquor to make a tincture. In a recent announcement, the FDA warned the public that there was a risk of adverse reactions between this herb and certain prescription drugs used for the treatment of cancer, transplant rejection, heart disease and AIDS, among others.

6. Borage – this potent herb has beautiful flowers that may be soaked in alcohol to prepare a powerful tonic that can boost your mood. The flowers and leaves may be used in tea preparations, eaten raw or soaked in liquor or wine to flavor the drink. The fresh plant provides a salty flavor with a cucumber-like smell.

7. Peppermint – this medicinal plant can be an effective tonic to promote better digestion. However, peppermint and any other strong mints such as pennyroyal must not be taken by women who are pregnant or possibly be pregnant. Drinks and foods that have fresh strong mint leaf can be harmful to the baby.

8. Pennyroyal – just like peppermint, pennyroyal is a great smelling mint which can be crushed and topically applied to the skin as a very powerful insect repellent. The leaves of pennyroyal can be crushed and topically applied to wounds as an antiseptic agent. It can also be used in tea preparations to tame upset stomach, however, do not over do it. The maximum recommendation is 2 cups daily. Consuming more than this recommendation may cause cramps and nausea.

9. Aloe vera – is a plant native to tropical Africa. This plant has spread worldwide as a first medicinal herb that provides soothing effects for scalds and burns. Aloe vera is best grown in a container so that it can be easily transferred indoors during the winter season.

10. Yarrow – for someone who's about to start a medicinal garden at home, yarrow is usually the top pick. This herb is a beautiful perennial plant that can serve a lot of different uses. Crushed yarrow flowers and leaves may be directly applied to scratches and cuts to reduce the chances of infections and to stop bleeding.

11. Slippery Elm – the inner back of this wonder herb can be ground and made into a nutrient-rich porridge-like soup. This can be an effective remedy for sore throat. In addition to this, the inner bark of this herb can be soothe irritations in the digestive tract.

12. Fenugreek – the seeds of this medicinal plant are nourishing and used to:

- Restore a dull sense of taste
- Freshen the breath
- Ease labor pains
- Ease painful menstruation
- Help in insufficient lactation
- Promote better digestion
- Help for late onset diabetes
- Darin off sweat ducts
- Treat inflammation and ulcers of the intestines and stomach

- Reduce blood cholesterol levels

- Inhibit cancer of the liver

- Encourage weight gain

13. Feverfew – is a plant which can be made into tea for the treatment of fevers, colds and arthritis. This plant is said to have sedative properties. It can also regulate menstruation. A feverfew infusion may be used to bathe swollen feet. It can also be made into a tincture for the treatment of bruises. Chewing about 4 pieces of leaves daily has been proven to be an effective cure for some migraine headaches.

14. Comfrey – an herb which contains allantoin. This substance is a cell proliferant which boosts the natural replacement of body cells. Comfrey is widely known for its ability to build strong teeth and bones in children. Comfrey is safer to use externally than internally. This wonder herb is used to treat a wider variety of health issues including the following:

- Varicose veins

- Eczema

- Sores

- Sprains

- Bruises

- Cuts

- Acne

- Severe burns

- Varicose and gastric ulcers

- Arthritis

- Sprains

- Broken bones

- Bronchial problems

15. Milk Thistle – this powerful herb can protect and improve the function of the liver. This herb may be taken internally to help treat the following:

- The effects of a hangover

- The growth of cancer cells in prostate, cervical and breast cancer

- Insulin resistance in patients suffering from type 2 diabetes who also have cirrhosis

- Increased cholesterol levels

- Liver inflammation or hepatitis

- Jaundice

- Gall bladder diseases

- Liver diseases

16. Wu Wei Zi – the fruit of this herb are reported to stimulate the central nervous system when used in low doses. In large doses, the fruits are said to depress the central nervous system while regulating the cardiovascular system. The seeds of this herb are used in the treatment of cancer. When used externally, this herb is used to treat allergic and irritating skin problems. Internally, this herb is used to treat the following conditions:

- Diabetes

- Hepatitis

- Hyperacidity

- Poor memory

- Insomnia

- Palpitations

- Chronic diarrhea

- Involuntary ejaculation

- Urinary disorders

- Night sweats

- Asthma

- Dry coughs

17. Sage – the latin name for this herb, "salvia", means to heal. When used internally, this herb treats the following conditions:

- Menopausal problems

- Femal sterility

- Depression

- Anxiety

- Excessive salivation

- Excessive perspiration

- Excessive lactation

- Liver issues

- Flatulence

- Indigestion

When used externally, sage is used for:

- Vaginal discharge

- Skin infections

- Gum infections

- Mouth infections

- Throat infection

- Skin infections

- Insect bites

18. Turkey Rhubarb – this herb is popularly known for its beneficial and positive effect on the digestive system. Even children can take advantage of the beneficial effects of this herb because it is gentle enough. In low doses, the roots can serve as an astringent tonic for better digestion while higher doses may be used as laxatives. In addition to this, turkey rhubarb is also known to treat the following:

- Skin eruptions because of toxin accumulation

- Menstrual problems

- Hemorrhoids

- Gall bladder problems

- Liver diseases

- Diarrhea

- Chronic constipation

19. Ginseng – is one of the most highly repudiated medicinal herbs in the orient. This wonder herb is touted for its ability to promote overall health, and general body vigor. The roots of this amazing medicinal plant is used to:

- Treat insomnia

- Address lack of appetite

- Treat debility related to old age

- Boost resistance against diseases

- Reduce levels of cholesterol

- Reduce blood sugar levels

- Enhance stamina

- Promote secretion of hormones

- Relax and stimulate the nervous system

20. Evening Primrose - the young roots of this medicinal plant can be consumed like a vegetable. The shoots may also be eaten as a salad. The roots of this wonder herb can be applied to bruises and piles. The roots may also be made into tea for the treatment of bowel pains and obesity. However, the more valuable parts are the bark and the leaves which are made into evening primrose oil, which is popularly known to treat the following conditions:

- Alcohol-associated liver damage

- Rheumatoid arthritis

- Brittle nails

- Acne

- Eczema

- Hyperactivity

- Premenstrual tension

- Multiple sclerosis

21. Tea tree – even the aborigines have utilized the leaves of tea tree for medicinal purposes, such as chewing fresh leaves to ease headaches. The

twigs, and leaves are made into tea tree oil which has antiseptic, antibacterial and antifungal properties. Tea tree oil definitely deserves a place in every household medicine cabinet. Tea tree oil is widely used for the treatment of the following illnesses:

- Minor burns

- Nits

- Cold sores

- Insect bites

- Warts

- Athlete's foot

- Acne

- Vaginal infections

- Thrush

- Chronic fatigue syndrome

- Glandular fever

- Cystitis

22. Great yellow gentian – the root of this powerful herb which is used to treat digestive problems. It is also capable of stimulating the digestive system, gallbladder and the liver. When taken internally, it is used to treat the following conditions:

- Anorexia

- Gastric infections

- Indigestion

- Liver complaints

Chapter 4: Know the Ten (10) Most Common Herb and Medicinal Garden Mistakes and How to Avoid Them

Common Mistake No. 1: Not applying any fertilizers.

Once you have herbs and medicinal plants planted and growing, it is very essential to keep them growing healthy with the use of a light, all purpose fertilizer. Apply a compost tea once every week to give your herbal and medicinal plants a boost. Herbs and medicinal plants are going to be harvested a lot of times during the growing season. This only means that your plants will be need an extra boost in order to keep their growth cycle for an extended time. When applying fertilizer, make sure to keep the soil hydrated and not the leaves themselves along with the compost tea. This practice will be healthier for the plant and contaminations in the leaves will also be avoided.

Common Mistake No. 2: Not protecting the plants enough.

While the herbal and medicinal plants are known to be hardy and resistant to diseases and bug problems, they can still arise. A lot of times, herbal and medicinal plant gardeners are scared to employ any strategy to safeguard their plants. This should not be the case. There are a lot of homemade and organic controls that are safe to use for edible herbal and medicinal plants. Organic gardening begins before the plant is even in place. Good soil and beneficial insects work altogether towards a chemical free herbal and medicinal garden.

Common Mistake No. 3: Not watering the plants properly

The needs of herbal and medicinal plants are very minimal. While they are very easy to maintain and care for, these plants will be providing you with fresh harvest all season. Herbal and medicinal plants however require proper watering schedule in order to remain free from stress.

Herbal and medicinal plants should be watered in the early morning, if possible. In this way, the water will soak deeper into the soil without having to deal with any evaporation issue. Always keep the soil around the plant hydrated and never water over the leaves as this will only promote diseases and mildews. Good mulch is important for your herbs as well. This will keep the soil hydrated and may extend the time between watering. Avoid mulching right next to the plant's stem though as this may invite insects and other types of invaders to make their home.

Common Mistake No. 4: Not paying attention to the tiny details.

It is a must to watch herbal and medicinal gardens closely. You need to know what the plant should look like while it is healthy as this will allow you to immediately notice when a problem first happens. Keep an eye on any damaged stems, leaves and disturbed soil around the plant. If you notice that the stems and leaves are beginning to fade, turn brown or curl up, you will have became aware of the problem early enough to possibly save the plant.

Common Mistake No. 4: Spraying chemical compounds into the plants

Herbs and medicinal plants are usually rinsed and used fresh. They should never be exposed to any kind of treatment that may possibly be toxic or dangerous to those who would eat them.

Even if a product claims that it is safe to use around pets and people, you should look for the words safe for edibles. You cannot rinse a bunch of basil leaves with water and soup prior to using. There are a lot of ways to keep ahead of the problems that may require the application of chemicals. Weed on a regular basis, watch the plants closely for any insect infestation and use natural fertilizers such as compost tea.

Common Mistake No. 5: Allowing the flowers to turn into seeds.

Herbal and medicinal plants grow beautiful flowers. While a lot of these plants have edible flowers, it is not a great idea to allow the herb to flower early during the growing season. Once your plant flowers, this signals that its life cycle is about to come into an end. Your plant is growing a flower, then a seed, then it dies back for that particular season.

It is a better idea to keep any blossoms from forming in the first place. When you see a flower about to grow, just pinch the entire thing off. You will notice that the plant may become persistent. In such case, cut the entire stem or below the flower.

Common Mistake No. 6: overcrowding or planting incorrectly

It is common to purchase more plants that you can possibly grow in a given area. When purchasing your herbal and medicinal plants, read the plant tags that usually come with each pot. Keep an eye to the width and height of the fully grown plant. You can always grow a quick growing annual between the plants, if you do not prefer the look of mulch. It is always a good idea to underplant rather than plant the herbs too close to each other from the beginning. Over planting is a big waste for money as it will not allow your plants to grow a healthy root system. A sturdy root system will help them survive the winter and expand the next growing season.

Common Mistake No. 7: Not cutting back enough

Pruning is what makes a plant to grow fast and neat. Pruning an herb implies that you are actually harvesting the good tasting stems and leaves. If you omit pruning, the plant will only tend to grow taller on a few stems. The leaves will grow old, dry and fall off. This will result to longer stems without leaves, Pruning will also allow the plant to begin and finish its life cycle. By regular pruning, you are actually keeping the plant in its growing phase for as long as possible. It will keep the flowers from budding, promotes leaves and stems and keeps the plant producing for an extended period of time. Your plants will appear healthier and better, if pruned back on a regular basis.

Common Mistake No. 9: Growing the plants in the wrong environment.

Are you growing rosemary, a chalky and dry loving plant in a humid and moist area? Your plant will surely die off in about 2 weeks from wet feet. If you would like to grow plants in a shady area, go for plants that can tolerate less sun. The sun=loving plants will grow weak and pale from not enough bright sunlight daily. If you have neither too shady nor too sunny area, try planting in pots that can be rolled or moved to the optimal lighting conditions. It is not a matter of sufficient shading or sun but is just a matter of finding a way to be adaptable to what you already have.

Common Mistake No. 10: Choosing unhealthy medicinal and herbal plants

The very first chance you have to find the perfect plant is when you actually buy it. Search for healthy plants, bright in color, plenty of foliage and certainly not one egg or bug on it. Finding a single aphid means that there are a lot more that you cannot see, all awaiting for the perfect time to invade your other plants. Never have the sympathy for a weak looking plant, unless you have a lot of space to keep it isolated from your main garden area while you try to repair the damage. The effort and time to be spent in repairing an infested herb garden means wasted time. Take the extra step to look for the healthiest plants that you can purchase.

Conclusion

Thank you again for purchasing this book!

I hope this book was able to help you to know how to successfully grow medicinal plants and herbs at home.

The next step is to follow the step-by-step guide and see your plants grow healthier each day.

Finally, if you enjoyed this book, please take the time to share your thoughts and post a review on Amazon. We do our best to reach out to readers and provide the best value we can. Your positive review will help us achieve that. It'd be greatly appreciated!

Thank you and good luck!

Check Out My Other Books

Below you'll find some of my other popular books that are popular on Amazon and Kindle as well. Simply click on the links below to check them out. Alternatively, you can visit my author page on Amazon to see other work done by me.

Coconut Oil for Easy Weight Loss

http://amzn.to/1i5f45p

Essential Oils & Aromatherapy

http://amzn.to/1ouuZTx

Superfoods that Kickstart Your Weight Loss

http://amzn.to/1eyHdku

The Best Secrets Of Natural Remedies

http://amzn.to/1gmHd7y

The Hypothyroidism Handbook

http://amzn.to/1emWfyR

The Hyperthyroidism Handbook

http://amzn.to/1kqLQCp

Essential Oils & Weight Loss For Beginners

http://amzn.to/Q83bFp

Essential Oils Box Set #40: Thyroid Diet & The Beginners Guide to Medicinal Plants

Top Essential Oil Recipes

http://amzn.to/1lSrhSC

Soap Making For Beginners

http://amzn.to/1fkmYwr

Body Butters For Beginners

http://amzn.to/1fWjwJe

Homemade Body Scrubs & Masks For Beginners

http://amzn.to/1jjLRIO

Carrier Oils For Beginners

http://amzn.to/1sbqUQP

Natural Homemade Cleaning Recipes For Beginners

http://amzn.to/1izDB2m

The Beginners Guide To Medicinal Plants

http://amzn.to/1vSujr6

The Beginners Guide To Making Your Own Essential Oils

http://amzn.to/1piUNSB

The Beginners Alkaline Miracle Diet

http://amzn.to/1sDVaVE

Essential Oils Box Set #40: Thyroid Diet & The Beginners Guide to Medicinal Plants

Thyroid Diet

http://amzn.to/1piW2RY

Essential Oils Box Set #1 (Weight Loss + Essential Oil Recipes

http://amzn.to/1qlYWWP

Essential Oils Box Set #2 (Weight Loss + Essential Oil & Aromatherapy

http://amzn.to/1qlYWWP

Essential Oils Box Set #3 Coconut Oil + Apple Cider Vinegar

http://amzn.to/1oIFZJw

Essential Oils Box Set #4 Body Butters & Top Essential Oil Recipes

http://amzn.to/1jSxURJ

Essential Oils Box Set #5 Soap Making & Homemade Body Scrubs

http://amzn.to/RAvJYo

Essential Oils Box Set #6 Body Butters & Body Scrubs

http://amzn.to/RAvSel

Essential Oils Box Set #7 Top Essential Oils & Best Kept Secrets Of Natural Remedies

http://amzn.to/1gvsRCq

Essential Oils Box Set #8 Homemade Cleaning Recipes & Essential Oil Recipes

http://amzn.to/1gxFAVb

Essential Oils Box Set #40: Thyroid Diet & The Beginners Guide to Medicinal Plants

Essential Oils Box Set #9 Essential Oil and Weight Loss & Carrier Oils

http://amzn.to/1jmcEPP

Essential Oils Box Set #10 Hyperthyroidism Manual & Hypothyroidism Manual

http://amzn.to/1nHgJU4

Essential Oils Box Set #11 Carrier Oils for Beginners & Coconut Oil for Easy Weight Loss

http://amzn.to/1nHfy6X

Essential Oils Box Set #12 Essential Oils Weight Loss & Essential Oils Aromatherapy & Natural Homemade Cleaning Supplies & Top Essential Oil Recipes & Carrier Oils
http://amzn.to/1nHfy6X

Essential Oils Box Set #13 Superfoods & Essential Weight Loss & Essential Aromatherapy & Body Butters & Soap Making
http://amzn.to/1nUds6v

Essential Oils Box Set #14 Weight Loss & Apple Cider Vinegar & Body Butters & Homemade Body Scrubs & Coconut Oil for Beginners
http://amzn.to/1i1qYOd

If the links do not work, for whatever reason, you can simply search for these titles on the Amazon website to find them.